The

Low Sodium

Diet

JOAN JONES

i

The Low Sodium Diet

Copyright © 2018

ISBN: 9781977036490

Warning and Disclaimer

Every effort has been made to make this book as accurate as possible. However, no warranty or fitness is implied. The information provided is on an "as-is" basis. The author and the publisher shall have no liability or responsibility to any person or entity with respect to any loss or damages that arise from the information in this book.

Publisher Contact

Skinny Bottle Publishing

books@skinnybottle.com

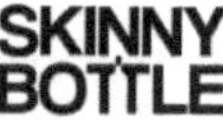

Dedication

I want to dedicate this book to my wonderful mother who never ceases to amuse me with her teasing of my writing on the walls of our house when I was a child, and to my amazing husband whose love and patience inspire me during many long hours of writing.

Joan Jones

Joan Jones is a Freelance Online Copywriter whose professional career began in 2015. She is a member in good standing of AWAI (American Writers and Artists, Inc.) and The PWA (The Professional Writers Alliance).

She has been awarded several articles and promos, some of which have been published.

Joan also worked at The Ohio State University (Health Information Services in Students Health), and The Ohio State Medical Center Department of *Nephrology* (medical science that deals with the science of kidney). Within the Department of Nephrology, she assisted *in the processing and shipping of biological samples*; and made phone calls reminding patients of their doctor's appointments.

Seeing the behavior and lethargy of kidney patients was her first exposure in recognizing some of the *symptoms and effects* that the intake of sodium can have on our bodies.

She has volunteered at The Mid-Ohio Foodbank, to inspire recipients on how to make healthy foods choices. On her websites: www.iwriteforhealth.com and www.platterenjoyment.com, she reveals her true passion for caring about matters concerning health, and how to live an abundant life!

In her writing, she gleans from the experiences of having worked as an Administrative Assistant and Secretary. She has had over twenty years' experience working for corporations like Rockwell International, Cedar Rapids, Iowa; The Coca-Cola Company Atlanta, Georgia; attorneys at law firms; and the Pre-Trial Office, U.S. Federal Courthouse in Columbus, Ohio.

She attended The Columbus State Community College.

A Matter of Quantity

*A*stronomical! **...** is the word for the level of documented cases of individuals who are at risk, or exposed to many diseases, including high blood pressure, and diabetes, as a result of the **amount** of their **sodium intake**, either consciously or unconsciously (maybe when dining out, or at relatives or friends).

Exotic Salt Shakers

So what's that tiny, cute salt shaker doing on our tables? They come in so many vibrant colors, shapes, sizes, and **exotic containers**; from wood to ceramic, and crystal ... they're so easy to pick up as souvenirs when we've run out of ideas, or our airplane is on the runway, and almost ready to take off!

We've been conditioned into thinking that it really doesn't matter *how much* salt we sprinkle on; we believe it's not going to make *much of a difference*. And having it as one of a central theme on *our dining tables*, a custom that's almost "as old as the hills," defeats the purpose of lowering our intake, especially when we could just as easily store it away in the pantry.

Water Retention Intensified

Salt stimulates water retention in the body and, *when eaten in excess*, raises the pressure of your blood; so if you have high blood pressure, your meds (diuretics) may not work as effectively as when you're on *a low sodium regimen*.

This can be a struggle for many considering the fact that it is included in everything popular that we consume; such condiments as ketchup, mustard, mayo, pickles-just a few. But because it is an indispensable component in the *culinary kingdom*, it's here to stay! And with good reason, it undoubtedly improves the flavor of the mouthwatering edibles we crave.

For centuries this mineral has been recognized for its satisfying qualities and values, and any great chef would be absolutely lost starting off the day without it in the kitchen.

Quantity is the Basis

It is quite a consolation to know that sodium is *not forbidden* for our consumption, but *quantity, quantity, quantity* could be the echo in our minds! "What should my optimum intake be?" Health experts have the answers. The best we can do is *glean from their expertise*, derived from intensive research, and practices, as they reach out to the world with their discoveries and conclusions; to provide us with excellent health and life-changing choices.

A Slow Approach

Slowly *cutting down* on the measure we consume can make a major difference in our overall health. But what is **"SLOWLY"**? For some of us it's a vague word in this context that might mean eliminating one salty habit a day; for others, it could be just cutting the amount in half for a while, but eventually avoiding it altogether, as may seem reasonable. Isn't *freedom of choice* an amazing thing? We've heard the term **"slowly"** so often that it has become superfluous; and may even be *occasionally* annoying, especially when it boils down to our eating habits, **a deeply sensitive topic**!

Consult Our Health Care Professionals

We're not ignorant of the truth that **not every method works** in the same manner for everyone; that's the reason **we consult our healthcare providers** to get a crystal clear understanding of what is meant by a **low sodium regimen** for you as an individual, and how to get started, with a new approach to your eating patterns.

Your doctor may need to know the **details** of what, how often, or where you eat; and what medications you're currently taking. He can then determine a safe and sound solution for you.

A low sodium regimen can transform our lives, and free us from deadly diseases and poor health. The **number one cause** of high blood pressure is **no longer a secret**; it is the consumption of too much salt!

Guidelines in Milligrams and Grams

Many clinical research professionals have concluded that people with high blood pressure should consume less than 2,300 milligrams (2.3 grams) of sodium per day. Others with other medical conditions might be instructed to consume significantly less—1500-1800 daily.

Quite often, especially on labels with small print, **milligrams** are often mistaken for **grams** when abbreviated; but the **contrast** is remarkable. I thought it might be helpful to point this out, particularly when thinking about the elderly, or people with impaired vision.

One very important thing to always keep in mind is *"per serving."* The amount of sodium stated on the label is only for *a specific serving size*; so when we change the serving size, we change the amount of sodium we're consuming.

Just imagine one teaspoon of **refined salt** contains about 2,300 milligrams (**2.3 grams**) of sodium, **exceeding** the daily requirement for many people!

Shun the idea of adding salt to food **during cooking** or before eating. Tasting before adding salt to your meals, and encouraging others to do likewise, is a habit that could be practiced and be beneficial. Bona fide studies have shown our taste buds may adapt to the depletion of sodium in our foods sooner than you may think possible.

Over-the-Counter

You'll observe that many over-the-counter medications, such as cough or sinus, contain a staggering, *high concentration* of sodium; so always check your labels, and find options that don't jeopardize your health, especially when you're on prescription medication.

The content of sodium listed on the label is alarming. Many healthier options are on the market and are easier to find now than several years ago. More than likely you're sure to find them in health food stores, and sometimes in regular grocery stores who don't want to discourage receiving business from people who are health conscious.

Your **healthcare provider** is one of your best friends and should be the source of valuable knowledge to ensure you're given dependable care for your medical concerns or anxieties.

Not Like an Addiction

By the way, some people have agreed that cutting down on salt is not, **by any means**, the same as withdrawal from a drug addiction. On the contrary, the comparison between the two is almost absurd, but drives us to *ponder the comparison*, and be tickled or challenged!

That's why I'm so hyped up and inspired about this topic, to persuade us to recognize that it takes just a tinge of "***discipline***" (that dreadful word) to escape *so many* health risks.

Compelled by Loss

But the highest motivation for writing about this topic comes from having lost my maternal grandmother when I was a very young child. She was the victim of a stroke, as a consequence of high blood pressure, and eating **highly salted foods**. She was not fortunate enough to be informed of the **valued alternatives** that we're so familiar with in this century.

She was only in her early fifties when she was suddenly snatched from her family and friends.   I savor exceptional memories of her great affection for everyone; and vividly recall sitting on her lap, feeling secure and well loved; and also her unforgettable, delicious cooking and presence in the kitchen where the aroma of food was inviting!

The list of the pleasures we enjoyed as a family is amazingly long. She was a "***one-in-millions***" treasure to everyone who had the privilege of knowing her.

Encouraging, New Technology

But this is not only about my grandmother, it's for you and me; *we now have the know-how* and wisdom that, when applied, make our lives so much better, ensuring our longevity and wellbeing; and I believe that's what most of us look forward to; we do care! And best of all, we **no longer have to agonize!**

Reliable Stats

According to the ***Center for Disease Control (CDC)***, 400,000 deaths each year are attributed to high blood pressure; and that about ***90% of Americans from two years old and upward*** consume too much salt; so, reducing salt intake would be an expert choice, to deter the occurrence of several thousands of deaths that occur annually.

The ***CDC*** also has a ***detailed listing*** of foods and their sodium content. Their principle is to save lives and protect people.

Strategies in Place to Reduce Sodium Intake

To defend the population against excessive intake of salt, sodium, blood pressure, hypertension and cardiovascular disease (CVD), strategies are being enforced by **FDA regulations** and suggested by the **Institute of Medicine,** such as*:*

- Educating the public by campaigning to increase awareness that links high blood pressure and hypertension **to the consumption of sodium.**
- Making dietary counseling by physicians and other healthcare providers available individually. Studies indicate that with focused counseling, a reduction in sodium intake can be more effective.
- Labeling foods was ruled by the **National Labeling and Education Act** in 1990, but measurements of **milligrams,** as opposed to grams, are not always easy to read, particularly for the elderly or vision impaired public. However, a concerted, voluntary determination by food industries, including restaurants to reduce sodium in their packaged product, is **the most critical resolution.**
- Policies established for **food purchasing policies** by government, and also in the private sector, should hold companies responsible for their promises to **significantly** reduce the inclusion of sodium in packaged foods.
- Following **FDA** guidelines, to **alter** the ranking of *"generally regarded as safe"* (GRAS) is recommended, as suggested by the **Institute of Medicine.**

A dogged attitude is looming on the part of the general public to drive more alertness in the planning of government agencies, such as the **FDA** and the **USDA** to accelerate the process of enforcing more stringent regulations for use by the food industries to drastically lower as suggested by the **Institute of Medicine.**

A Prediction

It's ***worth looking into*** the reality of what scientists predict: that by 2025, sixty percent ***(60%)*** of Americans will have high blood pressure! This awareness is becoming more intensified, and ***new medical research and strategies are in place*** to satisfy requirements and regulations that will meet the needs of millions in this country.

Progress in this endeavor is the reassurance that all is not lost; a *worthwhile mission in medical researches continues* that will impact the lives of millions who are hopefully anticipating ***long-awaited breakthroughs.***

Subtle Inclusion

The strange thing is, so many people are dying simply because they're unaware that *a high sodium diet is the culprit,* and because of ***the subtlety of its inclusion*** in almost every food we eat, it goes undetected or overlooked, and continues to seize front and center stage as the "subtle menace" that inflict many of us.

You might appreciate these simple and tasty tips for eating less salt!

- Replace with seasonings like ginger, chili, paprika, cumin, lemon, and real lime juices; herbs like basil, cilantro, dill, thyme, oregano, and rosemary. *Dried herbs and sauces may contain sodium*; notice the label.
- Try leaving out the salt when cooking; instead, you can try a low-sodium ***salt substitute*** (be sure to connect with your healthcare provider if you're taking medication).
  Himalayan salt seems to be gaining recognition.
- Avoiding products like stock cubes, and soy sauce (super salty) can really make a remarkable difference.
- Even labels on bread and cereals should be checked; some brands may contain a lot more than essential.
- It's also worth it to request less salt when eating out; it's not an imposition on restaurant policies since people are becoming more

aware of the need to eliminate it from their eating regimen. And, the good thing is, ***many restaurants will oblige.***

- The new ***FDA*** voluntary sodium targets will allow food ***manufacturers and restaurants to lower the amount of sodium in their foods***, giving you the power to choose.
- Scientists advise that ***for a naturally healthy person, 6g daily*** is all the salt needed for the normal functioning of the body.

Thankfully, herbalists and nutritionists have comfortable, *centuries-old* traditions of using certain ***herbs and vitamins*** as practical and likable substitutes; and this is quickly becoming the norm. People are changing their lifestyles, desiring more promising ways to live longer without undue concerns about their sodium intake.

Relevant Links

www.cdc.gov

www.ncbinih.gov/pmc/articles/PMC36112540/

11

Use of Cherished Information

Here are many advantages!

- ✓ *Use* canned beans labeled "no salt added" or "low sodium"
- ✓ Chicken or turkey breasts without the skin
- ✓ Low-or reduced-sodium cheese (e.g. natural Swiss cheese)
- ✓ Canned fruit packed in water or 100% juice, *not* in syrup
- ✓ Low-sodium, or "no salt added" ***ketchup***
- ✓ Unsalted Popcorn

POPCORN! I'd probably have to add just a tad. Pure, unsalted butter, canola oil, can be a tasty, viable replacement for sodium in your popcorn. Boxed varieties for microwave popping are notoriously laden with it.

Consider Himalayan Salt

H*arvested* from the Himalayas and known as the purest salt, it is now revered as *a superior alternative* and is rapidly taking its place on the table, instead of *refined table salt.* *Some* of the reasons Himalayan salt is so popular is that it *boasts many medicinal results*:

- ■ *It* controls the levels of water within your body
- ■ Regulates the pressure in your blood vessels

- Aids in absorption of nutrients in the intestinal tract, supplying the body with sufficient energy
- Promotes vascular health, bone strength, and respiratory function
- Prevents muscle cramps
- Regulates healthy sleeping patterns
- Wards off signs of aging
- Supports your libido

Since Himalayan salt has been sheltered from the earth's pollution as a result of being shielded by layers of snow and ice over the course of several million years, studies have revealed it has gained credence and is *deserving of our scrutiny,* and hopefulness.

Additionally, according to some sources, it is chockfull of nutritional values and essential, natural minerals, which ***may help to reduce*** anxiety and balance the levels of your blood sugar. It is also a useful detoxifier that may remove certain metals that might be trapped in the body due to human exposure to air pollution, living close to a mine; or drinking fluoridated water *that is believed* to contain lead, mercury, aluminum, arsenic, and radioactive waste material.

The plentiful hype and reasons seem to justify the need to ***try something new!*** And, add to the pleasure of its consumption. Many people ***(especially women)*** think that the color of Himalayan salt is appealing and pleasant!

Relevant Links

www.webmd.com

www.healthyandnaturalworld.com

www.livemint.com

www.rd.com

A Vital Nutrient

Although we've got to be cautious about how much sodium we daily consume, it is a nutrient that we need to survive; not a conflicting idea, when we welcome a strong **balance** into our regimen.

Endurance athletes are mindful that they desperately need it to replace sodium lost during competitions and high-level preparation workouts. They experience rapid water evaporation from the skin at each event.

We need sodium for our muscles to contract, to enable communication to the brain; and it is necessary for the functioning of the heart. Wow! How much more **vital** can it be to our health?

We're advised that adults should not exceed a 2300mg daily requirement; fewer when possible!

The pros and cons of the consumption of sodium are astounding-**we don't have enough,** *so we're lacking in some area of our bodily function;* **we have too much**, the same thought applies; but to eliminate confusion, a health professional should definitely be consulted to ensure that we're on the right path. And once we're at ease with our choices we'll be well on our way to peace of mind.

The **_www.heart.org_** suggests that 75 percent of the sodium in the American diet is from added salt in processed foods. This is because food manufacturers can get away with it?

Since it seems like most of what we purchase from food manufacturers and sellers is processed, the art of _**home-grown foods has infiltrated our country**_. People, more than ever, are growing produce in their backyard and are conscious and confident that they are well able to choose the quality of what they consume. Many are doing a flourishing business selling their crops.

And while even naturally grown foods contain some salt, to a degree, that could be the one that our body needs; and for people who grow their own foods, they have an advantage to live by.

The importance of knowing that a lack of sodium is dangerous, and may result in dehydration to the body in extreme temperatures, cannot be overlooked. When properly expelled from the body, sodium is normally nontoxic.

Not having enough can cause disorders in areas that affect good nutrition; so a safe guideline to follow is to consume _**from 2,400-3,000mg per day**_.

Relevant Links

www.fitday.com

www.heart.org

Foods High in Sodium? Fresh Routines - Adopted

To boost our *watchfulness of what we put into our mouths*, let's take a brief look at **some foods** that health professionals validate as high in sodium; some of these **we'd never suspected**, yet research has shown that it's prevalent in them, too. This listing is in order of popularity (or in *your* own order), and craved when ravenous! Imagine consuming these in large quantities! It's the cause of **Hypernatremia** (high-sodium level in the blood) in so many people:

- Pizza, especially meat pizza
- Salty snacks (you know the ones; so beautifully **packaged**)
- Hot dogs – a **blockbuster** treat!
- Processed cold cuts like salami, ham, pastrami, Bologna
- Spaghetti and the high-sodium sauce that accompanies it
- Macaroni with cheese
- White rolls
- Cooked rice when seasoned
- Processed cheese
- French fries (now some restaurants will hold the salt for you)

- Potato chips (there are many on the shelves that are lightly salted, or unsalted)
- Salad dressings like ranch, blue cheese; and other heavy, creamy varieties

Yet, so many reputable grocery *stores carry **low-sodium varieties*** of most of the above-listed items! They can be found in health stores and grocery stores as well; in every state across our country, and the world. Many imported goods are compliant with the standards of low sodium in foods.

Detection is Sometimes Difficult

Sometimes it's not always easy to detect the amount of sodium in foods simply by taste since many foods that don't taste salty can still be high in sodium; so caution should be taken to check labels for content.

Eating too much sodium is the main cause of high blood pressure and excessive fluid in the bloodstream. Swelling of ankles and feet, known as ***edema***, has been the consequence of overindulgence in sprinkling salt on meals, or adding too much salt during cooking, or eating out at restaurants. Other health disorders can occur, like heart, liver, or kidney failure because of high sodium intake.

Discretion

Judgment is yours; but how can you be ***discreet*** when you've eaten these most of your life? The amazing news is that *uncomplicated* means are now available, *more than ever before!* Experts and researchers in the medical and nutritional fields have painstakingly paved the way for us; and to our gratification, we can now guiltlessly make choices that are *not even "far off"* from unhealthy choices we've made.

They've learned how to ***adapt the foods*** we treasure and eat daily, ***to suit our palate*** so that we can enjoy them to the fullest, experience new explorations in eating, and live longer in the process.

We're urged to eat fresh foods like fruits, veggies; and meats that have not been injected and manipulated with saline solutions and sodium nitrates.

An Acquired Taste

We have been enlightened to the reality that our **taste for salt is acquired**. Fortunately, based on the findings of this research, we can safely conclude that this knowledge affords us the ease and flexibility to decrease the use of sodium, and surprisingly discover, that our taste buds have *(almost miraculously)* **adapted!** So, before long we'll not feel like we've been deprived of salt.

What a triumph this is for many sufferers of the *maladies we tolerate*; since there are ample possibilities with which to familiarize ourselves-by way of **clinical findings**; sensible food choices; and a determination that allows us to grasp control of what means so much to us-continuous, abundant health!

Hypernatremia is the medical definition that explains the condition of having too much sodium in the bloodstream. In mild cases, there may not be a cause for undue concern. Although sodium is a *necessary element* in our bodies, a balance must be maintained for our optimum health and welfare.

Relevant Links

www.healthline.com

Elaine K. Luo, MD

19

Symptoms and Causes of High Sodium (Hypernatremia)

Recognizing the symptoms of hypernatremia is the first step in being treated for the condition. Some symptoms are fever, diarrhea, vomiting which causes dehydration from the loss of fluids; excessive sweating; muscle spasms, or mental confusion.

These may be as a result of the medications you're taking, such as diuretics, or not drinking enough fluids, or you may have a kidney disorder. Older patients seem to be the ones most at risk, and in many cases, these symptoms are not detected as hypernatremia.

Diagnosis and Tests

To diagnose the symptoms of hypernatremia your doctor will have to take blood and urine tests to determine the cause. The condition can develop quickly or slowly over a period of time, and based on the speed of the fluid and sodium balance in your body. Close monitoring is necessary to ensure a safe and successful recovery.

When symptoms are mild simply increasing the fluid intake helps; but in acute cases, fluids are given intravenously into your bloodstream. This is always done promptly.

Generally Encouraging Outlook

However; the outlook for hypernatremia is usually good when detected at the onset and underlying problems are cared for and regulated.

Relevant Links

www.emedicine.com

www.healthline.com

www.livestrong.com

www.merckmanuals.com

Prevention of High Sodium

It's all too easy to shake salt onto our foods when the salt shaker is on our tables; keeping it in the pantry might help to eliminate our salt intake. The consumption of salt in American diets exceeds more than 50% the suggested amounts. And high blood pressure is the number one cause of excessive intake of sodium which can further result in kidney failure and **_hypernatremia_**. The **_National Kidney Foundation_** advises that one teaspoon **_per day_** of salt is the ideal proportion for the average body. These guidelines for eating are profitable:

- ✓ Fresh meats contain natural sodium and are preferred over packaged ones. You can tell that the sodium level is too high in a product when it can be kept for weeks without spoilage. This is certainly a red flag for you to consider.
- ✓ Select fresh fruit and vegetables; their natural sodium is very low, so are canned or frozen fruits.
- ✓ Choose frozen vegetables labeled **_"fresh frozen"_** and do not contain added seasonings or sauces.
- ✓ Whenever your shop, make checking every label for sodium content a routine in products like apple pie where it's hard to detect because the sugar level is very high.

✓ Many Spices and seasonings do not contain salt, for example: garlic powder, onion powder.

✓ Cottage cheese is a product that tastes less salty than it really is.

✓ We do acquire a taste for less salt over time, within a matter of a few weeks. But after this period has passed you'll find that everything you used to enjoy containing high sodium content will now taste much too salty.

✓ When planning to dine out, visit the website of your restaurant. There should be a listing of the sodium content of their dishes; you also have the option of requesting no salt in your foods.

Hypernatremia (high sodium in the bloodstream) can result from a lack of fluids, especially in the elderly. Drinking the amount of water, juices, and extra fluids throughout the day is one way to help combat high sodium levels but is even more critical during illness.

Elevated levels of sodium exceeding 150mEq/L in the blood, warrants *the attention of your healthcare provider.*

Another way to avoid high levels is to have your **blood tested** for abnormally high readings. The normal range is 135mEq/L. Levels should not be below 110mEq/L, or the chance of a seizure might be likely (according to **Medline Plus**).

Not adding more salt to your meals is a plus since most of what we eat is already infused with much more salt than the allowable amounts for a healthy functioning body.

Solutions Injected into Foods

Fish and other seafood are *sometimes* treated with *sodium solutions* that prevent spoiling; meat and poultry are sometimes injected. These can be avoided whenever possible.

Packaged breakfast, lunch, and dinner and other processed foods account for most of the sodium we consume, like in processed cheeses, cold cuts, salty snacks. Dining out in restaurants is convenient, but you can **make your**

requests known by preferring items that are not precooked, for example: steaks, vegetable salads, and others.

Rinse the sodium from canned foods like beans, corn, peas and other vegetables. According to the ***USDA*** after ***draining and rinsing,*** foods lose as much as two to nine percent (2%-9%) of their sodium. That's an impressive reduction that really helps when you purchase canned foods frequently.

The consumption of fresh fruits and vegetables throughout your day cannot be overstated for enjoying optimum health and energy and preventing the onslaught of a high sodium level.

In place of salt introduce fresh herbs like basil, thyme, rosemary, tarragon, curried powder, nutmeg, cinnamon; unsalted onion and garlic powders.

It can help to avoid consuming these high-sodium foods:

- Pasta sauce
- Vegetarian baked beans
- Pancake mix
- Pan pizza
- Cottage cheese
- Instant chocolate pudding
- American cheese singles
- White bread
- Low-sodium vegetable juice
- Bloody Mary mix
- Reduced-calorie Caesar dressing
- Canned green beans

Consult Your Healthcare Provider

Before using ***salt substitutes*** that contain potassium, talk to your doctor if you're taking medication; it may be threatening to a patient with diabetes or kidney disease.

Relevant Links

www.prevention.com

www.kidney.org

Symptoms and Causes of Low Sodium (Hyponatremia)

Studies have shown that insufficient amounts of sodium in the body, known as **Hyp_onatremia,** is caused by excessive fluid in the bloodstream, and may be the cause of low energy, headaches, irritability, vomiting, fever; malfunctioning of the kidney or liver; or an underactive thyroid. ***A health practitioner*** can determine whether symptoms are chronic and are the result of an underlying cause, or whether they only occurred within a few hours.

Rapid Loss of Sodium

The condition is deemed a ***critical medical emergency*** *when* loss of sodium in the bloodstream ***is rapid.*** But clinical researchers have shown that the prognosis for hyp_onatremia is *typically a good one,* especially when detected early.

Other Symptoms of a low sodium regimen may include congestive heart failure; frequent urination, and heavy perspiration; all of which cause fluids to collect and ***dilute sodium*** that is necessary for optimum functioning of the body.

Additionally, according to ***WebMD***, the symptoms of ***hyponatremia*** include restlessness, fatigue, muscle spasms, and confusion of the mind.

While it is *a necessary mineral* that regulates and sustains the balance of fluid; controls blood pressure flow, and stimulates a natural performance of the nervous systems, it also aids in synchronizing the operation of all the physical organs.

"Flooding"

Drinking water is basic and essential to life; however, excessive quantities, or ***"flooding"***, so named by *some health professionals*, reduce the sodium content in the blood, and the consequence is dehydration, which is detrimental ***when a higher content of sodium is necessary,*** as in the case of hyponatremia.

Taking antidepressants, pain medications, or diuretics, can severely contribute to incessant urination and sweating. ***Your health care providers*** are willing to guide you through the journey to determine what the most advantageous course is for your needs, by calculating the levels (***low*** [0.3g or less] ***medium*** [0.3-1.5g] or ***high*** [1.5g or more]) of sodium that is individually suited for you to ingest. Always connect with them first.

They can test you to determine the following:

- ✓ Low levels of sodium and amounts of electrolytes and minerals
- ✓ Urine content
- ✓ Low sodium in someone who has no symptoms; a basic metabolic panel can identify this.

People who are most likely to be at risk for having low sodium in the blood are:

- The elderly—whose sense of thirst is likely to decrease
- Those using diuretics or antidepressants
- High performance, athletic competitors
- People on a low sodium regimen
- People living in warm climates

Relevant Links

www.webmd.com

29

Prevention of Low Sodium

Drinking the **correct** amount of water is basic to avoid **hyponatremia (low sodium**), but especially during exercise. Athletes particularly are at a higher risk, and should also include drinks that contain electrolytes. If your body is exposed to extreme heat, extra attention should be given to ensure an adequate balance in your intake of fluids.

A nutritionally balanced diet should be eaten regularly to keep a strong equilibrium between food and liquid.

The Difference

Low sodium content in the blood is defined as **hyponatremia,** which is in **contrast** to high sodium levels, or **hypernatremia.**

When hospitalized, in critical care situations, and subject to receive fluids intravenously that replenishes their supply of sodium, people are sometimes prone to be a patient of **either one or both** of these.

Some Sources of Low Sodium

- ✓ Kidney disorders
- ✓ Disease of the liver
- ✓ Heart problems, or congestive heart failure
- ✓ Disorders of the adrenal glands
- ✓ An underactive thyroid
- ✓ Taking water pills (diuretics)
- ✓ Serious vomiting, or diarrhea
- ✓ Taking certain medications, antidepressants, or pain medications
- ✓ Dehydration

Tests You Can Take to Avoid Low Sodium

Your doctor can test your blood and determine low sodium levels. In cases where no symptoms are present your doctor can request a **basic metabolic panel**, which may pinpoint low sodium levels, even when a patient shows no sign of a low sodium diagnosis.

You're losing too much sodium when your blood sodium level is low and the level of sodium in your urine is high. You may also have too much water in your body, so your body is reacting to a loss of sodium.

To determine the amount of sodium in your urine, if your levels are abnormal, a **urine test** will also be run, so your doctor can arrive at a conclusion as to the cause of low sodium in your bloodstream.

Athletes are cautioned to drink the amount of water that's safe during workouts and to also drink other beverages that have electrolytes to replenish the sodium that may have been lost from sweating. A guideline to follow is to drink **three liters per day**.

It's advisable to maintain a balance in the amount of water and electrolyte your body absorbs so that you can avoid having low blood sodium; however, **rapidly** drinking too much water is not advisable.

Restoring Fluids

One of the ways to restore lost fluids is by drinking water, or beverages that contain *electrolytes,* and are either low in sodium or have none. These can be helpful in the following situations:

- ✓ When lost through vomiting, urination, or diarrhea.
- ✓ If you have a fever
- ✓ When you're at a high altitude in states like Colorado
- ✓ When you're pregnant or breastfeeding
- ✓ When the climate is warm

A helpful indication that you're well hydrated is when the color of your urine is **pale**, not orange colored.

It is also recommended that stability in hormone levels and adrenal glands be observed and maintained.

Relevant Links

https://draxe.com/hyponatremia

www.medicinenet.com

www.webmd.com

www.healthline.com

www.emedicinehealth.com

Tasty Foods Low in Sodium ... Spells Relief!

Before we delve into the blessings of these seemingly innocent edibles, let's consider a couple things: it's no surprise that eating on a low sodium regimen **could be tricky**, since we may defeat 0the purpose by *overindulgence*; if you're on a *low-sodium diet, quantities* should be limited to between 500mg and 1500mg *daily*, **according to the FDA.**

Consistency in checking nutrition facts on labels of the foods you purchase is of utmost priority when you're hunting for the finest foods; your firm judgment can be our guide—after all, you, your family, and friends deserve the best, which excludes excessive sodium in you meals!

This is not an exhaustive list by any standard, but here we go!

- Almonds
- Cashews
- Ginger
- Salmon
- Shrimp
- Asparagus

- Bananas
- Grapes
- Chickpeas (also known as garbanzo beans)
- Green Peas
- Chicken
- Eggs
- Milk
- Oats
- Limes
- Oranges
- Red Beef
- Broccoli
- Tomatoes

Fresh and frozen vegetables are nutritionally the best, but dieticians advise that if canned vegetables are chosen, they should be low in sodium, or thoroughly rinsed to remove excessive sodium.

This list almost covers everything we eat daily, although there are others, like exotic, imported fruits, vegetables, and meats from around the globe. Many of them are labeled but some need to be researched to determine the levels of sodium they contain; but we don't want to deny ourselves good foods with insignificant differences in the quantity of sodium, which might be the case with imported items.

Workable - Treatments for Low Sodium

There are several possibilities for treating low sodium levels (***hyponatremia***) before the condition escalates and is unmanageable. The underlying cause of a deficiency in sodium in the body is usually connected to dehydration, kidney failure, or an underactive thyroid.

Other factors that can contribute to hyponatremia are the use of recreational drugs or consuming high amounts of water. Other contributors are antidepressants, analgesics, and diuretics. Huge amounts of fluid loss due to severe diarrhea and vomiting may be responsible for the onset of this condition.

Hormonal changes may also be another cause of low sodium levels, according to a study by ***Mayo Clinic.*** "Depressed levels of the thyroid hormone, which is responsible for controlling the body's metabolism and other functions of the body, and malfunctions of the adrenal gland, which is a critical part of the body's sodium, potassium and water regulation mechanism, may give rise to hyponatremia" (***Mayo Clinic***).

These activities can deter the critical nature of this condition:

> ➤ Immediate action

> ➤ Lowering the amounts of fluids you consume

> ➤ Treating underlying conditions, like kidney or heart disease

> ➢ Infusing intravenous (IV) solutions
>
> ➢ Taking medication for symptoms such as headaches, nausea, seizures

Postponement of Care

Signs of *hyponatremia*, or an abnormally low sodium level, should be *treated promptly* and your fluid intake carefully monitored. Immediate attention to the problem will result in the stability of sodium levels in the bloodstream. This method has been proven to be the most effective.

Your healthcare provider must be informed of any medications, including diuretics and drugs that you're taking in order to proceed with an accurate treatment; you may need to change the medications you take.

An isotonic saline solution administered intravenously helps stabilize the levels of sodium.

Reduce your water intake, so as to increase the sodium levels. Drinking less water prevents dilution and will raise the concentration of sodium in your blood flow. A sports drink containing electrolytes is beneficial when you're exercising from running and perspiring.

Some salt should be added to your foods. Consider eating foods that are low in caloric content, such as vegetables, fruit, salads, and sandwiches, while repeatedly checking the levels of your sodium.

Relevant Links

www.draxe.com

www.livestrong.com

www.mayoclinic.com

www.reference.com

Simple Shopping-Detection Guide

This is a simple guide to have on hand that will assist you as you choose your foods. It can be taken with you as you shop and shouldn't take long to get used to. As you continue to shop, especially if your purchases are about the same each time, you'll have no problem purchasing meals based on your list of the foods that meet your needs. Like most things, before too long, it'll become routine and a valuable habit.

Although your label reads **unsalted or no extra salt has been added**, there may still be some naturally occurring salt in the food. It only means that none was **added** during processing.

A **sodium-free** label on your item means that there's less than 5mg of sodium per serving. These should be eaten in abundance, a safe choice.

Very low sodium means that you get 35mg or less of sodium in each serving.

Reduced sodium assures you that there's at least 25 percent less sodium in every serving than in the typical variety.

Low sodium means that there's 140mg or less sodium in each serving. Small amounts eaten occasionally might be sufficient to satisfy your craving.

A label that reads **_Light in sodium_** will contain 50% less sodium in every serving.

A banana has only 1 milligram of sodium; they're practically sodium free! There's a very small margin of sodium among fruits and vegetables, and that's the basis for treating ourselves with generous amounts of these.

A valuable thing to remember is that you don't have to be **_under the supervision of a doctor_** to decide to eat right; so why wait until you're endangered, by unknowingly consuming sodium in amounts that may not conform to healthy eating habits?

Many people have been amazed to find out how much they were actually ingesting, as opposed to what they **_thought_** they were. It's so enlightening when we wake up, "pinch ourselves", and start off on the right track ... it's really a new beginning!

Foods with a 5% Daily Value (DV) or less is preferred over a Daily Value (DV) of 20% or more. This will be seen on the Nutrition Facts label.

Imagine eating these foods every day!

- ✓ A bountiful supply of fresh fruits and vegetables, like bananas, grapes, peaches, apples, oranges
- ✓ Canned fruit that's packed in 100% juice or in water
- ✓ Spinach, carrots, broccoli, collard greens, tomatoes
- ✓ Low sodium vegetable juices
- ✓ Frozen, unsweetened fruit
- ✓ Unsalted, canned vegetables or those low in sodium

Many foods contain **_seasoning packets_**, it's advisable to use only a small portion and use on other portions later; this will lessen the content of sodium that you consume.

Instead of seasoning packets, you can also use herbs and spices and unsalted powdered seasoning; ginger, chopped garlic, onions, red and green peppers, limes, and lemons.

When cooking pasta it's best to not add salt. This can also apply to grains, oatmeal, popcorn, and packaged cereals.

Breads that are multiple-grain, or whole wheat and low in sodium, are the healthiest choices. Some are very high in sodium.

Fresh meats are naturally the best, but others contain sodium and are sometimes injected with solutions to prevent spoiling. Continue checking your labels.

Nuts, Beans, Meats

- Skinless chicken and turkey breasts
- Eggs
- Dried peas and beans
- Unsalted nuts and seeds
- Fish (especially salmon that have been wild caught), or shellfish
- Canned beans with no added salt or are low in sodium

Vegetable oils like olive, peanut, avocado, and canola not only liven up your foods but adds rich color and is appealing to your taste.

Unsalted butter can be used sparingly because of its flavor; light mayonnaise and salad dressings, such as French and others like a vinaigrette dressing containing apple cider vinegar and any of the good oils. They can be boosted with some onion and garlic powder and a hint of ketchup or mayonnaise.

Milk, Cheeses, Yogurt

- Low fat (1%) milk
- Fat-free milk
- Cheeses low in sodium (or reduced) like Swiss cheese
- Soymilk
- Yogurt with low sodium, or fat-free

Relevant Links

www.drugs.com

Low Sodium during Your Pregnancy

Apart from its ability to support energy and hormone production, salt is unquestionably lifeblood for general health. It is important in the development of the brain in unborn babies, their intelligence, memory, language.

Studies have shown that babies with low sodium in their bloodstream due to a low salt intake by mothers during pregnancy are more like to be underweight at birth and are vulnerable to various health problems as they grow and develop.

Meticulous Care

But it's important to keep in mind what is the precise amount of sodium for you to ingest. ***Your health caregiver*** is able to direct you to the best choice for you and your baby.

A low birth weight can be the result of eating a diet low in sodium; and the likelihood is strong to increase your chances of developing headaches, tiredness, or hypertension, which put stress and pressure on your blood vessels and heart. A healthy daily guideline for sodium consumption is 200 to 500 mg for maintaining a significantly healthy body.

Eating Suitably

Introducing herbs into your meals while reducing the amount of salt is a great start to caring for the well-being of your unborn child. Fresh fruits and vegetables, low-fat milk, chicken, lean meats are advisable. Avoid cold cut meats that contain sodium nitrates, such as bologna, salami; canned soups and foods, and foods that contain MSG.

Also, low-sodium **bacon** that does not contain sodium nitrate is widely available (most of us love the taste of bacon). Several varieties of nuts, chips, and crackers are readily obtainable in many grocery stores, and especially health food stores to suit your palate and ensure that you have a safe and good pregnancy.

When dining out you can request that no salt be added to your meals.

Your nerve, muscles, and all other organs need salt to perform their natural functions. During pregnancy your body's amount of fluids increases. Sodium helps to stabilize these functions which, if insufficient in the bloodstream, can be a major cause of miscarriage or stillbirth.

Too much sodium can cause swelling and bloating of the ankles, feet and other parts of the body. And we've all felt uncomfortable at some time after consuming meals that were laden with salt, even when not pregnant, so just imagine what it'll do for a woman during pregnancy; the effects are multiplied.

Labels

Checking the nutrition labels on condiments, especially ketchup, barbecue sauce, and certain salad dressings might surprise you. It's worth your time to observe the "mg" content in each one. Cereals, and bread, too, can be a delicate choice on your part. You'd not expect to find as much sodium in these. The "per serving" size for cereal is usually one cup, but who's completely satisfied with just one cup, so finding the brands that contain less sodium gives you the edge when it comes to quantity consumption.

Another point to remember is that something that ***doesn't taste*** salty is no indication that it isn't. So looking at those labels will steer you in the right direction.

Even controlling our intake of sugary drinks like juices, soda, hot chocolate mixes, is advised during this important time. They, too, contain a degree of sodium, so a careful selection is the key.

Eating at Home Whenever Possible

Whenever possible, it's always best to prepare your own foods so you can manipulate how much sodium will go into it; but too often we as mothers become tired and that's the last thing on our minds unless relief from someone else is obtainable. Otherwise, just being careful with our shopping choices, and making wise selections when eating out at a restaurant, or elsewhere, requesting that salt is excluded from your meals, should be sufficient.

Using ***simple***, nutritional, low-sodium recipes is a blockbuster idea; there are hundreds online, also small recipe books out there that you can use and keep handy; even children's cookbooks can be quick and easy to use; since ***easy preparation*** is what you deserve!

Relevant Links

www.whattoexpect.com

www.healthybabycode.com

44

Low Sodium Diet in Nursing Mothers

This is one of the most important things that you may do for your baby, so being meticulous in the process is not being "fussy." Choosing a diet low in sodium should be your main concern, especially when it comes down to the effect it can have on the quality of your breast milk.

Having a balance in your sodium levels is positively related to assisting the transmission of impulses from your nerves, and also aids in contracting and relaxing your muscles.

When choosing your baby's food try to remember that a baby's kidney is unable to process sodium successfully. It is recommended that you purchase foods that are designed for babies. They are lower in sodium and try to not add salt to their foods.

True Incentive

Being on a low-sodium diet is an incentive to eat a variety of fresh fruits and vegetables since that is what's necessary to supply much of the nutrition your milk needs, although sodium does not appear to affect breast milk according to clinical studies. But keep in mind that it is also important to have the correct amount of fluids in your body to avoid dehydration, which might affect the quality of your breast milk. It's reasonable to have a drink of water or juice just before breastfeeding.

Imagine eating at least two servings of fruits and vegetables daily, along with poultry, lean meats, seafood, eggs, nuts, seeds and grains (wheat, rice barley millet, corn). This is a productive pattern to follow, especially when breastfeeding.

It's a good idea to consume milk and yogurt that are low in fat, to add valuable calcium, along with other protein-rich foods.

The experts advise that sufficient iodine should be a part of your daily regimen for the ideal growth of your baby.

Fluid Intake

Drinking too much water causes the body to retain fluids which may cause hypertension, kidney disorders, and other complications. Sodium works like a magnet to water and you'll find that you urinate more often than normal, and your heart has to labors hard to keep the body in balance.

One teaspoon of sodium per day or less is the maximum requirement recommended by most doctors.

Findings of Sodium Levels

Studies were conducted by ***The Department of Nutrition at the University of California*** in which breastfeeding mothers were fed different sodium levels, to show how it affects the milk. The mothers were given specific amounts at lunch, and the conclusion of the study proved that the milk was not affected, no matter how much sodium was consumed; the results ***were the same*** on different afternoons.

Relevant Links

www.modernghana.com

www.healthyfood.com

Low Sodium in Children

There seem to be widespread concerns among medical health professionals about children consuming excessive amounts of sodium in their meals. Obesity is now an epidemic which is being addressed more than ever. Fast food restaurants provide sodium in quantities that are much higher than the daily allowances for your child and approximately 80 percent of what children eat is laden with sodium, by way of processed foods. Reduction in the levels of sodium they ingest should be started at an early age to avoid obesity and hypertension.

Soft Drinks: The high consumption of soft drinks by children is also linked to obesity in children, and the threat of having high blood pressure and heart disease become greater.

Maintaining the ***proper levels of sodium*** is crucial for transmitting nerve signals, and supporting muscle contraction. A diet low in sodium needs to be in place, which will sustain the normal pH of the blood.0.00

Kidneys store sodium in your child's body when the level of sodium is dropped; then it is accumulated in the bloodstream, which may result in severe health disorders.

It's been recommended by the dietary guidelines of ***The American Heart Association*** that children ***up to three years*** old should ***not consume more*** *than* 1,500 milligrams of sodium daily; children *four to eight years* of age should consume *less than* 1,900 milligrams of sodium daily; from nine to 13 years old*, less than 1,200 milligrams*, and those *14 to 18 years* old*, less than 2,300 milligrams (2.3 grams)*.

When sodium accumulates, the blood volume increases; a high blood volume causes the heart to work intensively to pump the blood. This increases blood pressure and poses a risk for heart disease or stroke.

As we read the labels to regulate the sodium content, watch out for the ones that say "reduced sodium, or "light in sodium quite possibly may still have a high content of sodium. Avoid foods with more than 200 milligrams of sodium per serving (according to *the Mayo Clinic*).

Consulting with *your health care provider* and carefully reading the labels on food products is a foolproof way of determining that your child is consuming only the amount of sodium that is necessary to provide optimum health.

Relevant Links

www.livestrong.com

Low Sodium in the Elderly

The elderly who live in health-care or assisted-living facilities, or are hospitalized, are the most susceptible to low blood sodium (hyponatremia). This is present when the amount of sodium in your blood is unusually low or there's too much water in your blood. Lethargy, confusion, or change in personality, are signs of hyponatremia.

A history and physical exam should be initiated. In severe cases, seizures, coma or death may occur if not quickly spotted, assessed, and controlled.

Excessive water in the brain cells can cause headache, nausea, and confusion.

Therapeutic approaches are accessible, such as intravenous isotonic saline used in severe cases. Malnutrition and limited cognitive function are often factors in determining the cause of hyponatremia.

This is more widespread among the elderly since they're understandably taking medications for conditions that cause them to be vulnerable, such as:

- Frequent urination from some drugs
- Anti-seizure medication
- Underactive thyroid or adrenal glands
- Pneumonia
- Urinary tract infections

- Some antidepressants
- Certain Cancers
- Slow functioning of the heart, kidneys, or liver

It may also be necessary to change medications that may alter your sodium levels when receiving treatments for hyponatremia to treat an underlying disease. This may also include modifying the amount of water you drink or changing the amount of salt in your diet.

Patients with hyponatremia and extracellular fluid have congestive heart failure or liver disease; and the kidneys will hold on to sodium to try and alter the surplus of fluid, which results in a decrease of sodium in the urine.

For treatments to be effective in improving sodium levels, focus on the underlying cause of hyponatremia and it is ***critical to know the patient's extracellular volume status.***

Relevant Links

www.medscape.com

www.ncbi.nlm.noh.gov.com

www.mayoclinic.org

Heart Failure and a Low Sodium Diet

Having to live with a condition like heart failure can be quite overwhelming at times but recovery can be forthcoming by reducing the levels of your daily intake of sodium. It is found in many foods, especially salt. This mineral causes your body to retain a lot of water which floods your bloodstream and causes heart failure.

When sticking with a low-sodium regimen your blood pressure is under control, your breathing is easier, and swelling of your feet or ankles is eased.

Your mains course meals can be enjoyable and flavorful:

> ➢ Select fresh fruit and vegetables
> ➢ Stay away from cured meats, canned or marinated vegetables, pickles, seasoned croutons, cheeses, and salted seeds.
> ➢ When dining, order your salad dressing on the side, but use a small amount.

When cooking, try to use fresh ingredients or foods with no added salt. The recipes that mean the most to you can be adjusted to meet your need for a low-sodium regimen, and in some cases, you may need to **discontinue the use of certain foods**. It's encouraging to note that salt can be removed from any recipe, except the ones that may contain yeast.

There are multiple items to choose from for *your main course* meals; with some caution, you can eat without undue concern about your sodium intake when dining out:

> ➤ Select foods like grilled, broiled, or roasted meats; fish or shellfish; chicken, turkey.
> ➤ Select plain vegetables, potatoes, pasta, and noodles.
> ➤ You may want to check with your server about their low-sodium choices and the preparation of the food.
> ➤ Stay away from restaurants like buffet restaurants that have no special preparation guidelines.
> ➤ Casserole dishes and sauces and gravies tend to be high in sodium; it's best to stay away from these.
> ➤ Eat fresh fruit ice cream, sherbet, plain cakes, gelatin, and ices.
> ➤ Ask that your food is prepared without salt or monosodium glutamate (MSG).
> ➤ Avoid fast food restaurants.

- *Consult with your healthcare provider about using a salt substitute*; it's usually not a great idea while you're taking medication.
- Avoid packaged foods like canned soups (*use low-sodium canned soups*) and vegetables; frozen dinners; entrees, instant cereals; gravy sauce mixes, and puddings.
- The frozen entrees that you purchase should contain no more than 600 milligrams of sodium; even less is better. Always check the nutrition facts on the package.
- Fresh, frozen, or no-added-salt canned vegetables can be used. But always thoroughly rinse your canned vegetables to eliminate most of the sodium that was added.
- Instead of using blends of spice and seasonings that contain salt, trying using low-sodium ones. Nothing else has been added to the *onion and garlic powders*—they're sodium free and add excellent flavor to your meals.

There's no need for your foods to taste bland because of the symptoms of heart failure. Too many amazing *alternatives are available* in health food stores and now, many grocery stores, to shop for the right items that add flavor to your foods and keep you on the right track.

Here are some sodium-free substitutes for seasoning your foods. Combine these ingredients in a small bowl and blend well. Spoon into a shaker, then store in a cool, dark place:

o   Two tablespoons dried savory, crumbled
o   Quarter teaspoon freshly ground white pepper
o   One tablespoon dry mustard
o   Quarter teaspoon cumin
o   Two and one half teaspoon onion powder
o   Half teaspoon garlic powder
o   Quarter teaspoon curry

A *spicy Seasoning* that can also add to the enjoyment of your food;

o   One teaspoon cloves
o   One teaspoon pepper
o   Two teaspoons paprika
o   One teaspoon coriander seed (crushed)
o   One tablespoon rosemary

Excellent No Salt Added Option:

o   Two teaspoons garlic powder
o   One teaspoon basil
o   One teaspoon oregano
o   One teaspoon powdered lemon rind or dehydrated lemon juice

An excellent guideline for your daily intake of sodium should not exceed 1,500 milligrams. And this should be the same for most people whether they have heart failure or not. Imagine how much good it can do for someone with heart failure!

+Here's a nourishing *breakfast* to start off your day:

- ✓ Fresh fruit
- ✓ Low-sodium cereal (hot or cold)
- ✓ Milk

A *lunch* suggestion:

- ✓ Lean roasted turkey on whole wheat bread with low-sodium mustard
- ✓ Raw carrot stick
- ✓ Applesauce
- ✓ Milk
- ✓ Vanilla wafers
- ✓ Half a cup of chopped, cooked, frozen or canned fruit
- ✓ Half a cup chopped, cooked, frozen or no-salt-added canned vegetables
- ✓ Half a cup of low-sodium tomato sauce
- ✓ Half cup pasta (noodles, spaghetti, macaroni
- ✓ 0Half cup rice
- ✓ Low-sodium crackers

A *dinner* suggestion:

- Grilled chicken, or fish
- Boiled potatoes
- Steamed fresh vegetables
- Tossed salad and low-sodium dressing

Snacks

- Fruit
- Walnuts or almonds
- Raisins
- Yogurt

Eating about five servings per day of these *bread and grains* can significantly improve your condition: Have six or more serving of these *breads and grains* daily: one slice of low-sodium bread; one small low-sodium roll; half of a low-sodium bagel.

These *sweets and snacks* can be enjoyed once in a while. Try to stick to your goal:

- ✓ Two and a half ounces of unsalted nuts
- ✓ One slice of angel food cake
- ✓ Half a cup low-sodium potato chips, pretzels, popcorn and similar snacks
- ✓ One tablespoon jelly or honey
- ✓ One cup sherbet, sorbet, or Italian ice
- ✓ One ice popsicle
- ✓ Three fig bars or gingersnaps
- ✓ Eight to 10 jelly beans; three pieces hard candy

Fats, Oils, and Condiments are necessary to flavor your foods; using the ones that will relieve your symptoms can be the best choice you make:

- ✓ *Use these as much as possible*:
    - o Vinegar
    - o lemon juice
    - o herbs and spices without salt
- ✓ *Use these only when necessary:*
    - o Olive and canola oils
    - o Low-sodium butter
    - o Low-sodium soups
    - o Low-sodium salad dressing
    - o Homemade gravy without salt
    - o Low-sodium catsup
    - o Low-sodium mustard
    - o Low-sodium sauce mixes

Relevant Links

www.webmd.com

Low Sodium in Diabetics

Some of us have wrestled with the idea of whether or not people with diabetes needed to lower their sodium intake in a huge way, yet most clinical studies and research validate the fact that a person with diabetes are ___under the same regulations and guidelines___ as others without it, where sodium intake is concerned. It is suggested that the average person can safely consume 2,300 milligrams (mg) of sodium per day, although people usually consume up to 6,000 milligrams of sodium daily.

Reducing your sodium does take a little time, maybe two to three months, since our taste buds tend to adapt easily to changes. Your choices of food and vegetables are numerous and are able to help keep you on the right path, but it's best to not add salt to your food before cooking, also avoid sprinkling on food just before eating.

Restaurants are Complying

Many restaurants will comply with your request to hold the salt on many of your favorite items, like steak, French fries, salads, and others. Some foods that are not cooked ahead of mealtime are practical options.

Nothing beats the desire, or ability, to prepare your own meals, or to have family and friends do it for us; however, we have quite a number of options available in the restaurant industry while we're away but want to continue on a regimen that is a safeguard to our health and wellbeing. The awareness in restaurants is prevalent

Selections for Food

Here are healthy selections with which you might already be familiar:

- Fresh fruits and vegetables
- Fresh meats, containing no salt or not injected with solutions to prevent spoilage.
- Skinless chicken and turkey breasts
- ***Read labels*** and select "low sodium", or "no salt". Levels less than 140mg per serving is acceptable.
- Care can be taken when purchasing frozen and packaged entrees; a safe rule to follow is that an entrée should not exceed 600mg of sodium per serving.
- Use a scant serving of salad dressing and condiments like pickles, olives, mustard, and ketchup; these are particularly high in sodium.
- Salt substitutes should be used according to the advice of your healthcare provider; the potassium level may be too high and can intermingle with medications that you may be taking.

Relevant Links

www.my.myclevelandclinic.org

Low Sodium for Weight Loss

Sodium seems to be the culprit everywhere we look, and it seems to be especially true when it comes to weight gain. Studies done by researchers seem to agree that sodium is related to weight gain and modifies the way fat is absorbed into our body.

Foods are now conveniently packaged, which makes it so much easier to "grab and go", especially in a culture where everything is done with high technology in mind. The constant rushing to have things done at a fast pace leaves no room for homemade meals or even simple ones. We just stick packaged dinners into the microwave and in a matter of seconds, the meal is ready.

Determining Quantity

Eating at *some* fast-food restaurants may pose another problem; it may be difficult to control your salt intake. Look at their food *online nutritional listing* **to determine the quantity** of sodium you should include in your diet. At least you'll have a guide as to your intake, and be able to adjust as you decide to change your eating patterns.

The milligrams of sodium we consume daily are astronomical and are usually twice the recommended amount. The finding is that men, on an average, consume 4,243 mg; and for women, the amount is 3,000 mg daily, according to ***Queen Mary University in London.***

Researchers have concluded that red fruit contains more anti-fat components, like phenolic compounds that regulate the fat in your genes, than does green.

Imagine the *amount of packaged foods we consume*, most of them laden with chemicals, are like ***magnets*** for fat cells! Consuming fresh foods and vegetables are a must for weight loss; foods cooked at home contain less sodium and you can control how much goes into it. Eating at restaurants can be a challenge; but you can request that no salt be included in certain items, for example, French fries, or on dishes that are not made ahead, like gravies and soups.

One great advantage to consuming quantities of fresh fruit and vegetables over time is that you see the results in your sleeping patterns, your skin becomes invigorated, and in other ways, on an individual basis.

A super breakfast

It gets you off to a great day start and eating a breakfast that is a good source of protein is an advantage. For example: poached, eggs with ***bacon*** (low-sodium, and containing no nitrates. This can be found at supermarkets); and a whole wheat biscuit.

Eggs contain choline, which is a nutrient found in meats, seafood, and greens, Choline attacks the genes that prompt your body to collect fat around your liver. The versatility of eggs is had to overlook; from making omelets to even incorporating cooked ones in salads; some people even like the idea of putting them into a veggie smoothie.

Greek yogurt

This is tasty with berries; fat burning smoothies—fruity or veggie, and will provide nourishment that ***your body craves*** to remain strong. The veggie smoothies provide faster more appetite-curbing and muscle building benefits at a faster rate. And it takes a matter of seconds to whip these up.

A Pitcher of Antioxidants

Another prized idea for weight watching that's become really well-known and practiced by many people is the habit of *setting out a pitcher* of your allowable water intake for the day, then infusing it with fruit like lemons, oranges or any citrus fruit. They're full of antioxidants, which "flush toxins from the body" (*World Health Organization*) and stimulates the fat-burning process.

Make yourself a *trail mix* chock full of protein, with a variety of nuts, seeds, unsweetened dried fruit, and bits of dark chocolate. Monounsaturated fats found in peanut butter provide you with a high percentage of protein and tummy-slimming benefits, including fiber.

Peanut butter

High in monounsaturated fats, it is also quite well-known to fight hunger and is a source of fiber, which boosts your metabolism; it also contains genistein, a compound that inhibits the genes that promote obesity. Check the label; it should read: peanuts, or peanuts and salt, no fillers such as sugar, palm oil, and other obscure ingredients.

Wild caught salmon

Heart-healthy omega 3 fatty acids promote the normal functioning of the heart including flexibility in heart rate. According to the *American Heart Association*, fish should be consumed at least twice a week, especially salmon, herring, black cod, mackerel, and sardine.

Wild caught salmon also supplies vitamin B12, B6; selenium which supports the immune system; phosphorus for energy; also vitamin D for strong bones.

It is harvested from oceans and rivers and feeds on natural food in its natural environment. It is also rich in minerals, potassium, and iron.

Eating fish often is a deterrent to strokes and heart attacks. Inflammation from heart disease is also reduced. It also lowers very high levels of triglycerides in the blood of people with type 2 diabetes.

Another advantage of eating fish is that it boosts your "good" *cholesterol (HDL)* level and your blood pressure can be better controlled so that your weight gain can be at a minimum.

Blood clots are needed for healing wounds; however if clotting is too quick, a blood vessel can be blocked, and this is critical. Omega 3s protect from this happening by producing red blood cells.

Fish oils in large doses have been used to treat *rheumatoid arthritis* that causes pain, swelling, and stiffness. Caution should be taken when taking large doses if you're taking blood-thinning medications.

The benefits derived from eating wild caught salmon and digesting omega 3s is insurmountable—from fighting cancer to healing eczema, supporting cognitive skills, and curing many other disorders. It will do us all good to make this a part of our eating standards.

Farmed Salmon

It has been researched and studied, and reports from the *Environmental Working Group* (EWGA) states that the crowding of salmon on farms poses a contamination problem, and may be associated with cancer-causing PCBs at high levels.

They are also fed processed food pellets and other chemicals to speed up their growth; also corn and soy, which is unlike what salmon would normally consume.

The problem of fish lice is a quite a dilemma since drugs that are used to kill them, can infiltrate the environment by polluting the oceans and rivers.

Imagine this, it has also been discovered that farmed salmon contain toxic chemicals and dioxins! Farmers have been accused of environmental issues such as promoting diseases in the oceans. Other issues such as the food content raise questions about chemicals and supplements that are being included in feeding the fish that add a pink color to farmed salmon.

Farmed salmon contains over 1,900 mg of ***unhealthy omega-6s***.

It seems like the choice is clear as far as the propriety of research is concerned: eating wild caught salmon is the healthier for you, especially if you already have a pre-existing condition.

Health food stores generally carry wild caught salmon and you're more likely to find the best selection there. Packages should read "wild caught" and not words like "organic", "imported", or "natural". These are words that mean "farmed", but they are disguised to mislead the customer.

Beans such as garbanzo (or chickpeas) and others, pureed with herbs and/or spices, with onions and garlic, in extra virgin oil, or canola oil, to your desired consistency, are used as dips for low-sodium crackers and chips.

Adding a ***salad to each meal*** with a little vinaigrette will speed up the weight-loss process by helping the body absorb fat-soluble nutrients. Arugula, kale, collard greens, watercress are the top choices according to nutritionists and healthcare professionals. Avocados are rich in monounsaturated fats that block the build-up of belly fat; it can also curb hunger pangs for several hours.

A rapid loss in weight may be the result of a reduction in your salt intake. Sodium causes your body to retain water, and your body weight to increase, according to ***Diets in Review.*** A substantial amount may be lost initially, but the pattern will not continue if you assume the old habit of eating.

Foods labeled "no salt added" can even have saturated fats in them, which defeat the purpose of your sodium regulation. As you regularly continue to ***manipulate*** your sodium intake you'll find that you can achieve a reasonable loss in weight. The ***ADA*** endorses DASH to comply with the standards for helping to lose and maintain an ideal weight.

Moderate exercise, of course, is a must along with sodium reduction to maintain a healthy body.

Relevant Links

www.eatthis.com

www.livestrong.com

www.healyeats.com (farmed salmon)

https://eatwildsalmon.com

Low Sodium Diet for Vertigo

Eating right can be sometimes demanding while enduring **vertigo,** but to be in peak health simple measures can be taken to achieve this goal, upon which your wellbeing depends. Sickness can hit us as a result of poor eating habits and not getting the nourishment our body needs. The right diet for you may not be the same for everyone else, so it's best to consult your healthcare provider to determine the right choices.

Symptoms

Vertigo is difficult to comprehend unless you know someone who is a patient or you have experienced it. The symptoms are dizzy spells, unbalanced sensations with the feeling that you're being pulled to one direction. Headaches, sweating, nausea, sudden jerks of the body, ringing in the ear and abnormal eye movements are all symptoms.

Diet Matters

To prevent vertigo from erupting, managing our good intake is vital to have a strong balance of body fluids. Rejecting certain foods can help relieve the symptoms that are present in your body resulting from vertigo. So here are some foods that can be harmful to you if you have vertigo:

- ❖ ***Foods high in sugar***
  It's been proven that foods *high in sugar* affect fluid balance. Candy, sodas, donuts, cereals with a high sugar content, chocolate, can cause flare-ups of vertigo. Try eating sweet fruits instead.
- ❖ ***Foods high in salt*** counteract the natural balance and regulation of fluids in your body. A low sodium diet should be your choice by avoiding foods like crackers, pretzels, potato chips, and similar snacks.
- ❖ ***Nuts and Seeds*** are very high in tyramine and may be linked to migraine headaches in vertigo patients.
- ❖ Tyramine is also present in ***Meats and cheeses***. It would be a helpful plan to avoid items like Swiss cheese, brie, cheddar and ricotta; also pepperoni, and many other sausages.
- ❖ ***Certain Over-the-Counter Medicines*** such as antacids, aspirin, contain extremely high amounts of sodium and should be replaced with options from a health food store or grocery stores that also carry medicines that are lower in sodium. Some of these may cause water retention and affect the balance of electrolytes in your bloodstream.
- ❖ ***Nicotine*** can be harmful to your body, decrease the blood supply to the inner ear, and compress your blood vessels. You may also experience hypertension which can activate vertigo, as a result of ***nicotine*** in the body.
- ❖ ***Yogurt is high in calcium*** and may be the reason for a flare-up of vertigo when large quantities are consumed.

Recommendations for Eating

- ✓ Try eating plenty of fish
- ✓ Foods that are rich in magnesium can help reduce vertigo symptoms. Vertigo has been linked to magnesium deficiency. Green leafy vegetables, certain nuts, seeds, and beans are high in magnesium.

- ✓ Eat whole grain bread instead of white bread
- ✓ Eat plenty of fresh greens
- ✓ Drink plenty of water, especially if the weather is hot, or you're exercising
- ✓ Avoid trans-fats
- ✓ Introduce veggie juices whenever you crave drinks that are high in sugar.
- ✓ Staying away from caffeine when possible; it can stimulate migraines and vertigo.
- ✓ Wines should be avoided because of the inclusion of tyramine

You'll be managing the symptoms of vertigo when you eat the right foods. Be consistent with your plan to take action, and merge it with a regular exercise routine. Consulting with *your health care provider* is the safest way to ensure that you're receiving optimum guidance to control your vertigo.

Dehydrate Inner Ear by Reducing Sodium

Not to be confused with the middle ear, accumulation of fluids in **the inner ear** should be taken seriously and a physician consulted, who may, after running tests, prescribe water pills to relieve symptoms such as tension in the ear, ringing, or dizziness; and sometimes loss of hearing. If you have an acute case, you might be advised to use antibiotics. However, it is easily treatable when cared for at the onset.

Food Consumption

Normally, foods are not known to cause ear problems, but evidence shows that some foods may induce or exacerbate the symptoms of ear disorders. Consuming too much salt, like in potato chips, pretzels, French fries, soy sauce, processed, packaged foods, and meats adds to the danger of further infecting your ear.

It's best to reduce your intake of foods that are plentiful in sugar, such as candy, pastries, cookies; beverages like soft and energy drinks, and sweetened fruit juices. Healthy options are available in grocery stores and health food stores. Making these at home, when possible or convenient is a fantastic choice.

Soft Drinks

Homemade soft drinks and sodas are becoming the rage, and contain no damaging preservatives or additives, so you can control and infuse them with your favorite fruits and flavors.

Not a Serious Concern

Although it is not uncommon to discover growths, tumors or infections in critical cases, these are not popular.

One of the only means to dehydrating your ear is by being on a low-sodium regimen. In **Chapter 5** of this book, you will find safe recommendations for eating hearty nutritional meals that your palate will welcome. The **Simple Shopping detection Guide** will not only help you to lower the fluid levels in your ear but also give you a perspective on healthy eating in general.

The reason for including this section is to state that, unknown to some people, even having fluids in the ear can be a result of excessive sodium in our diet and to emphasize the importance that having a balance in our sodium intake does positively *affect our entire body*

Relevant Links

www.todaysdietician.com

Loyola Medicine: Inner Ear Fluid Imbalance

Cochlear Fluid Labs, Washington University: Fluid in the Ears

Mayo Clinic: Meniere's Disease: Treatment and Drugs.

www.healthfully.com

www.livestrong.com

Low Sodium to Reduce Swelling

Many of us have witnessed others with ***edema,*** or have had the experience of having swollen ankles or feet. Conditions like pregnancy or liver disease, having a diet high in sodium, or taking certain medications may account for edema. Identif0ying and treating the underlying cause and cutting down on sodium in your diet can help keep the body from retaining excess water, which may help in reducing the swelling.

Eat plenty of fruits and vegetables that are naturally low in sodium will increase you're the likelihood of reducing the swelling in your feet and ankles. Fresh, frozen, and canned fruits are usually sodium free. Exclude frozen vegetables that have sauces and other additives that include extraordinary amounts of sodium.

Meat and beans are high in protein. Having a low level of protein in the blood may be the cause of edema. Eat fish, and fresh meats and poultry that are not injected with solutions to prevent spoilage; levels of sodium are staggering in these items.

Dairy products are a beneficial source of protein, but some may contain too much sodium. Labels have to be checked to make sure the levels are low enough for your consumption. Some cheeses are too high in sodium. You may consider consuming milk and yogurt as suitable options for reducing swelling in your feet and ankles.

Keep the salt shaker away from your table and try to avoid adding salt during cooking or before eating a meal.

Condiments like ketchup, barbecue sauce, soy sauce, olives, pickles, canned soups, and others that are similar foods with sodium content should not be included in your diet for trying to reduce swelling.

Always connect with ***your health care provider*** to get answers for any questions or concerns that you might have about swelling of your ankles and feet, and especially the limits of your sodium intake, which is usually the core of these problems. You'll find that there are solutions when we try to follow the guidelines presented to us that help to improve our health.

Relevant Links

www.livestrong.com

Manipulate Weight Loss-Lower Sodium in Men

Making a decision as to **how much sodium** should be consumed is *not* always as *easy as 1-2-3*; especially when it adds flavor to your foods. It is even more difficult for people who are "on the go" and have limited time to get from one destination to another. Choices have to be made that will be beneficial to your overall wellbeing. You still have the option to select foods that are low in sodium by requesting them from restaurants and other places when dining away from home.

Just a Pinch

In many instances, we'd be surprised to find that *just a pinch* will do when preparing meals or dining out, but it has been ingrained in our cultures that more is always better. The thought of settling for less hardly crosses our minds. A change in ideas is fast surfacing, and more caution is being used when choosing foods that are lower in sodium. We realize that the difference in taste is not as significant as we'd thought it could be.

Fast foods pose a real problem where sodium is concerned as they have a high amount of sodium.

Grilled or Steamed Options

Choosing foods like salads and ***grilled or steamed food options*** instead of fried, can change the order of your eating habits and will be beneficial in the long run. Condiments are another thing; ketchup, barbecue sauce, mustard, pickles, mayo can be consumed lightly. Menus for fast foods are available online and list the nutritional content.

Fresh or frozen vegetables are a must. Canned vegetables tend to be salty and should be rinsed before eating.

Teenage Men

While young teenage men don't have to rigorously watch their sodium intake, it's a good idea to observe modifications suggested, to avoid having high blood pressure, or diseases that may be a result of overindulgence in the consumption sodium.

A recommendation by The Institute of Medicine (IOM) suggested the following consumption rate for adults per day:

- 1,500 mg for people ages 9 to 50
- 1,300 mg for adults ages 51-70
- 1,200 mg for seniors over 70 years old

However, the boundary for adults should not exceed:

- 2,300 mg (2.3 g) for a healthy adult
- 1,500 mg a day if your blood pressure is high or you have diabetes or kidney disease, black, or are middle-aged or older.

A Few Statistics

The Center for Disease Control (CDC) indicated that the average American daily intake of sodium was over 3,300 mg. It further states that 400,000 deaths each year are ***attributed to*** high blood pressure as a result of excessive ingestion of sodium.

Records from ***Statistics Canada*** have shown that Canadian men consume far more sodium than Canadian women.

Positive Strides

It could mean a positive transformation in our ***health patterns and total wellbeing*** if we adapt to ideas suggested by medical researchers and nutritionists:

- ✓ Limit snacks that are high in salt, like chips, crackers, popcorn. Many manufacturers now restrict the amount they include in their brands and these can be easily found in many grocery stores and health food stores.
- ✓ Select fresh fruits and vegetables and eat them in abundance.
- ✓ Try to avoid pickled foods since the concentration of sodium is intense.
- ✓ If you love canned soups, you definitely want to check the sodium content; it's unusually high.
- ✓ Pre-packaged foods are quite tempting and sometimes convenient but ***laden*** with sodium. For example: frozen dinners, mac and cheese, lasagna, meatballs; and many others. It can be challenging to find some that are ***as low*** in sodium ***as we'd like***, but they're available. Searching out the better ones is well worth a bit of extra time.
- ✓ Oh, **condiments!** Soy sauce, barbecue sauce, mustard, and pepper sauces. We can't afford to leave them out, but we can prefer to reduce them.
- ✓ ***Bacon*** (who doesn't like it), and other cured meats such as ham, salami, bologna, pepperoni, without the inclusion of sodium nitrates, can now be found in stores.

Taking the time to maintain health patterns is a rewarding venture that we'll cherish for many years and pass along to other generations.

A Natural Reaction

As we consume salty foods, sodium enters the body by way of the bloodstream. The volume of blood is increased, ***dehydration takes place*** and a hormonal reaction is stimulated, so drinking fluids will be the ***natural response***. Drinking fluids restores the stability of water in the body.

The choice that athletes who need to be certified must make prior to weighing in, or for confirmation before a bodybuilding competition, is to restrict sodium, food or fluids two days in advance.

Before Weighing In

When food intake is restricted for a couple of days before ***weigh-in,*** hunger takes over, but the body is able to adjust for the short period; however, health problems like irritability, lightheadedness, headaches, are likely to happen. During that time, water, protein, and glycogen will account for about two-thirds of the weight that you lose.

It is advisable ***not to restrict your water intake***, as this can be detrimental to the tissues in your body, which reduces the amount of urine that is expelled, causing water to generate a *significant loss of weight*. This affects the blood, organs, and muscles.

Studies have shown that men are more prone to consume a higher amount of sodium than women, which result in a greater presence of chronic illnesses; and it is shown that men in their thirties are the most likely targets. When approaching the age of 40, the intake of sodium seems to lessen, although elderly men over 69 tend to consume more than 3,000 milligrams of sodium on a daily basis. A ***safe daily consumption*** would be a maximum of 2,300 milligrams (or 2.3 grams).

Harmful Consequence

What seems to be a secret to most people is that our taste buds have a way of adjusting to sodium, and as we ***slowly eliminate it from our diet***, we'd be amazed to find that it's "not such a big deal" after all; we're still enjoying our foods, but with less sodium; and we have only reduced it from our meals. The only thing that happens is that we've now become tougher and healthier!

A high sodium level is a warning that you may be at risk for high blood pressure; it compels the body to retain water, which makes the heart work harder to drive blood through your veins and arteries; and your kidneys also have to work *just as intensely*, to rid the body of water.

Safer and More Appealing Selections

- Because bread is such *a craved staple* for many of us, when and if possible, choose whole-wheat bread over other bread, as it contains approximately a quarter less sodium; many others tend to be much higher and increase the levels of sodium in our bodies.
- When you're ravenous for fast foods, choose the ones lowest in sodium; check online listings of fast foods' nutritional standards and content of sodium.
- Canned foods, especially soups, seem to be one of the downsides to eating on a low-sodium regimen. When convenient, homemade is, naturally, the best choice; and many are super simple to make. But *even canned soups now come in low-sodium varieties* with meats and vegetables.
- *Label reading* is a must to determine how much sodium is in your foods, based on your guidelines. A *low-sodium* item may contain less than *140 milligrams of sodium* in a serving; the trick would be to adjust the *number of servings* you consume.
- Using herbs and flavorful spices is another satisfying discovery many people have made, and some have claimed that the taste for sodium has been lessened *to a point* that the craving is no longer present; *others are now using* Himalayan salt, which is becoming the standard for many.

More Benefits and Results of Studies

It has been documented in a study from *Nagasaki University* that when you cut down on your intake of sodium, your sleep becomes interrupted, so you spend less time making fewer trips to the bathroom.

Additionally, *UNC Chapel Hill* researchers have concluded that too much salt is damaging to your liver and that foods that are labeled "low salt" or "reduced salt" are worse than the other refined choices. Their moral is: "Don't eat processed foods."

The *American Heart Association (AHA)* advises that to "maintain normal blood pressure"; healthy adults shouldn't exceed 2,400mg of salt" in a day; although the body needs a certain amount of salt to control blood pressure; so stay within the safety limit of 500mg per day, and not take in more than that quantity.

While lowering your salt intake, you should be certain that you're also getting enough potassium, magnesium, and calcium; all of which have a valuable effect on the pressure of your blood and the risk of heart disease. Increasing your fruits, vegetables, protein, and dairy products is a great thing to do.

Always, *checking in with your health provider* is a blockbuster suggestion to meet your individual needs, and for the best possible guidance for keeping your sodium at optimum level!

Relevant Links

www.mensfitness.com

www.mensjournal.com0

www.healthyeating.sfgate.com

www.youngmenshealthsite.org

www.measkmen.com

www.humankinetics.com

Forty-Year-Old Female Normal Sodium Regimen

In considering the normal sodium for women who have reached the age of 40, we understand that *for most women* at that age it is much more of a challenge to adjust the taste buds to a better way of eating.

Sodium, naturally found in some foods, is vital to great health and assists with the functioning of your muscles and regulation of fluids in your blood cells. High quantities of refined salt (or sodium chloride), is an endangerment to blood pressure and triggers the development hypertension which can result in heart attacks or strokes. The risks are severely higher for women at forty and older.

Curbing the intake of your sodium can save your life, and as it has been noted, the craving for salt can easily adaptable when we realize that we can enjoy our meals with a significant decrease in sodium, while also incorporating herbs and spices in our daily eating habits.

The average increase in the consumption of sodium was 55 percent, from the 1970s to 2004, as a result of the *explosion* of processed foods, containing *too much* sodium.

So, the reality is that the consumption of sodium for0 a healthy forty-year-old female should be **2,300 milligrams (2.3 grams) daily** or less. But a safe alternative would be to consume **1,500 milligrams daily (according to the USDA) if your blood pressure is high.**

It is also recommended that, in addition, a daily consumption of **4,700 milligrams a day of potassium** be included, to efficiently aid sodium in regulating fluids and blood pressure levels.

Breakfast Time!

It's your first meal of the day and you can be excited about it knowing that you are consuming all the right things. Imagine oatmeal sprinkled with nutmeg, cinnamon, and some vanilla bean or vanilla extract; and flavored even more with pure maple syrup or honey! Cream of wheat can be flavored in the same way; whole wheat toasted bread; smoothies of any variety—veggie or fruity; yogurt with 140 milligrams or fewer.

Most instant breakfast cereals tend to contain added sodium; be watchful as you pick your options.

The versatility of omelet is so encouraging at breakfast time; so much can be safely added and so much can be left out. Vegetables like red and green peppers, onions, and low-sodium cheese, mushrooms, spinach, and others.

Lunch Time

Who's craving salmon fillet with herbs, served with couscous or brown rice; tenderly cooked, grilled chicken, or pork, topped with honey braised sliced carrots? Your choice of veggies is limitless.

A healthy low-sodium salad can contain some of these as well, including a non-creamy dressing since these tend to be high in sodium. It's **best not to add s0alt** to any of these. French dressings, or a simple oil and vinegar, are preferred choices.

Dinner Delights

Eating Pizza, using meats very low in sodium, and those that contain no sodium, or sodium nitrates, is obtainable; and vegetables of all varieties can be added Using low-sodium tomato sauces that can be purchased in health food stores, and even other supermarkets.

Zero-sodium flour can be found, too!   When or if time permits, easy recipes can be seen online and in recipe books that encourage low-sodium eating. Some restaurants conform to these standards as well, if you have no choice but to eat away from your home, or are simply always "on the go." Let's face it, pizza is irresistible for most of us; ***why deprive ourselves?***

Baked chicken, or salmon, served with honey glazed pineapple, or peaches, baked sweet potato. Unsalted tuna in a tortilla with veggies, plain Greek yogurt with a touch of mayo, a splash of fresh lemon juice, chopped onions, red and green bell peppers, extra virgin oil, and some freshly grated black or white pepper.   Add a pinch of Himalayan salt, and presto! How outstandingly luscious is that for your palate! ... That's not even mentioning all the health benefits you gain.

Snacks to Satisfy

Here they are! Homemade ***potato chips*** or store-bought, low-sodium ones that meet your guidelines are available. A-low sodium dip might be needed, or beans of all kinds pureed with fresh onions, garlic, a splash of fresh lemon juice, extra virgin oil to desired consistency and spices.

Grapes are easy to grab; fresh juicy apples, plums, berries of all types are easy picks.

Popcorn can be popped in canola oil and a drizzle of melted unsalted butter added at the end, or maybe lightly sprinkled with a pinch of salt; unsalted cashews in a blender with dates and formed into a ball.

If you're not allergic, unsalted, no-stir ***peanut butters*** are in stores and can be a satisfying snack with honey on whole-wheat, low-sodium bread. Other butters like cashew and almond are also tasty and filling.

Up-to-Date Substitutes

There are *so many safe food discoveries* that have been made in the industry pertaining to **low-sodium selections,** that there's no need to settle for less than the best for ourselves, families, and friends. We can now **substitute** our foods to improve our health and fitness.

To **neutralize the sodium content in your body**, drink more water and consume **potassium**. Foods such as oranges, spinach, sweet potatoes, acorn squash, avocados, and whole grains are rich in potassium.

If you're on medication, **always consult with your healthcare provider** before making changes to your diet. He can also prescribe a potassium supplement.

Relevant Links

www.livestrong.com

Enjoying a Low-Sodium Breakfast

It's been a *widely-accepted fact* that your breakfast is your most important meal. You want to kick off the day with a nourishing start! But it seems that many breakfast items are laden with sodium, and we tend to absorb more salt than necessary. Most people already consume exorbitant amounts, which is the cause of high blood pressure, kidney problems, and many others.

Taking a turnaround and transforming the way we eat breakfast can meaningfully alter the amount of sodium that enters our bloodstream. We want to stay within the limits of about 1,500 to 2,300 milligrams (2.3 grams) of sodium every day.

The best picks are:

- *Whole Grains* are a great fiber source, and also curbs your appetite so that you're not famished before your next meal; the advantage is that their sodium content is low.
- *Fruits and Vegetables* are certainly low in sodium and are great sources of vitamin C, potassium, and also fiber. Apples, melon, oranges, berries, grapefruit, yogurt, are all excellent breakfast choices. Tomatoes, kale, or spinach can be easily added to quiche; additionally, bell peppers, mushrooms, onions, parsley, cilantro, spinach.

- ***Smoothies*** are quick, not just for people on the run, but for everyone who just wants to drink something instead of sitting down to a meal; and they fortify the body in a remarkable way.
- ***Nuts*** of all kinds can be added to smoothies for extra flavor, thickness, and added protein.
- ***Eggs***, also low in sodium but high in protein. The flavor of eggs can be enriched with the use of herbs, and vegetables, excluding salt. Small amounts of water can be added instead of milk to reduce the sodium content. Black pepper and paprika add color and flavor.
- ***Meat***: Decide to select meats, ***bacon***, sausage, and others that contain no sodium nitrates. Imagine, one strip of ***bacon*** contains 192 milligrams of sodium. So multiply that by a couple of slices and you've almost arrived at your daily sodium limit. But many people can settle for just a slice or two? Chicken or turkey may be better alternatives. But try to get the low-sodium kind and ***not deprive yourself*** of eating bacon.

Relevant Links

www.everyday*health*.com

A Lunch Low in Sodium

Let's think whole grain crackers, Swiss or mozzarella cheese, peanut butter, cashew, almond, and others! Lunchtime is not only a cherished time to socialize, but it's also a time to replenish our supply of nutrients after hours of having had breakfast, so we're ready to eat another hearty meal, and are conscious about our sodium intake. After we've decided to make the right choices, it easily becomes the norm and choosing is simpler.

- *Canned, low sodium tuna* can be found in many stores, and can be mixed with mayo, or Greek yogurt. Including onions, chopped celery, red and green bell peppers for added color and flavor makes this a nutritious combination. Low-sodium, whole wheat bread, supply you with a power-packed lunch.
- *Butters like almond, cashew, and peanut* are a great choice to have with a handful of raisins and a helping of fresh fruit.   They, too, have to be checked for the sodium content. Bananas, apples, grapes, strawberries are everything your body craves. Always depend on the advice of your healthcare provider.
- *Avocado* which supplies heart-healthy fats has become so popular. When combined with grilled chicken, turkey, finely chopped vegetables, and hard-boiled eggs, it makes succulent sandwiches.

- ***Garbanzo beans, or chickpea*** (when pureed it becomes hummus). Other grains can be pureed as well and added to salads. Quinoa (KEEN-WAH), kidney beans, and barley are all delectable choices.
- ***Salads and dressings*** are savored, especially when the best combinations ***suit individual tastes***. Instead of store-bought prepared dressings, a low-sodium choice of vinegar and olive oil can be preferred. Careful choices of cheeses, meats and pickled vegetables like pickles and olives can be added.

Always ***consult your health care provider*** to be sure you're following a healthy routine.

Relevant Links

www.everydayhealth.com

Indulge with Low-Sodium Dinners

What could be more stimulating than the anticipation of eating *a flavorful dinner?* Knowing that the food choices you're making to *lower your sodium* intake are the right ones, adds to the enjoyment of the meal. It's the last large meal of the day and we want to end the day "with a bang!" Here are some examples of mouthwatering, low-sodium meals.

Chicken fajitas: cooked in olive oil, onions, red peppers, chili powder, ground black pepper, paprika, cumin, oregano; enclosed in tortillas with finely shredded iceberg lettuce, guacamole, salsa, more onions, finely shredded, tomatoes, crushed garlic cloves, and coriander leaves.

Salmon: glazed with low-salt wholegrain mustard and maple syrup; oven-grilled on a tray,   with the skin on; with steamed broccoli or asparagus, or vegetable of your preference.

Steak: with melon and a low-sodium vinaigrette dressing, along with onions, parsley and combined with other vegetables, make a satisfying protein-filled dinner.

Turkey: roasted with herbs such as chopped, fresh thyme, celery stalk; minced garlic, and black pepper.

Lasagna Rolls: whole-wheat lasagna noodles Instead of ricotta cheese you might try well drained and rinsed tofu; minced garlic, baby spinach; crushed red pepper, olives, low sodium marinara sauce, part-skim mozzarella cheese, in extra-virgin olive oil. Pinch of salt.

Mushrooms: grilled Portobello caps stuffed with plum tomatoes, extra virgin olive oil,

part-skim mozzarella cheese, Kalamata olives, fresh ground black pepper, minced garlic, finely chopped rosemary, lemon juice; low-sodium soy sauce.

Relevant Links

www.bloodpressureuk.org

www.eatingwell.com

www.health.com

Managing Low Sodium in the Summer Months

It can be confusing that we can we can drink several glass of water in one day and still have a low level of sodium in the blood. But this is possible when you're taking diuretics to help control blood pressure. So though diuretics remove fluids from your body, sodium levels become depleted.

Hyponatremia which is a consequence of Low sodium levels in the blood poses a health drawback. So we've been admonished to stay fully hydrated in the hot weather by drinking water and other drinks that contain electrolytes.

Regularly connecting with your health care provider is the best way to be prepared for the summer months, which should be free from undue concerns about your sodium level and the discomforts of possibly having hyponatremia.

In some cases your health care provider may limit the amount of water you drink, or stop the diuretic, and may cause the normal level of sodium to rapidly return.

It's not always easy to observe all the workings of sodium in the blood. Diuretics can be cause of low sodium when the blood volume is low; so it must he treated when the volume is high. So being dehydrated could be the result of not sufficient fluids in your bloodstream. But low sodium levels need to be treated when you aren't hydrated.

Sodium attracts and brings water to your arteries and veins at the correct levels. If the sodium level is too low, the concern must be whether the volume of fluid is at the normal level.

If you're dehydrated and your sodium level is also low, prompt action should be taken to replace the lost volume, and the low sodium is normally corrected. But in cases where your blood volume is normal and your sodium is low, medications you take for depression, seizures, or recreational drugs may be the offender. An anti-diuretic hormone causes the retention of fluids in the kidney, and too much of this hormone is the cause of excessive fluids and low sodium.

When your blood volume is normal and your sodium level is low, the first course of action would be to restrict the fluid to lower than two liters or less per day, to control the dilution of water. But the underlying cause should be the focus, to determine whether the condition is hormonal or a side effect of the medication you're taking.

Another important fact is when you have low blood sodium and the volume of blood is overloaded resulting from heart, liver, or kidney failure, immediate action will be taken to give diuretics to restore the blood volume to its normal state, and at the same time, the sodium level will naturally return to its original state.

Relevant Links

www.foxnews.com

Marc Siegel, M.D. NYU Medical Center

Sodium Deficiency in your Pets

The only way to determine the amounts of sodium your pet should consume is by carefully gauging its health. Have **your vet thoroughly check** and evaluate for **alertness**, first. The canal of your pet's ears should be examined to see and feel any unusual lumps or redness due to inflammation, or if painful; odor of breath; smoothness and shininess of coat; frequency of bowel movement, and changes in appetite.

Levels of Sodium in Your Pet

The sodium levels in your pet's blood are regulated by a hormone produced in the adrenal glands called aldosterone, which alerts the kidneys to preserve and reabsorb sodium from the urine produced, which through its urine eliminates excess sodium in its body. These of diuretics for congestive heart failure can cause a low sodium level to be present.
Overuse of certain laxatives can also be the source of a sodium deficiency.

Safe Guidelines

This scrutiny will provide credible guidelines for preserving your pet's health, and you'll know how much sodium is best.

Food selection should be based on these factors to insure normal growth and vigorous development. Rely on the ***judgment of your vet*** to make the right choice. ***Keeping a log*** of the content of the food your pet consumes is of extreme importance; observing anything he might be allergic to.

Many reputable brands of pet foods and recipes ***low in sodium*** are available for you to make a sensible choice as to their nutritional content, and taste preference of your pets; this is ideal for maintaining the normal ***blood pressure of older dogs***.

Hyponatremia and Fluid Retention

Sodium deficiency ***(low)*** in dogs and cats, also known as hyponatremia, may ***also*** be described as a ***high level*** of sodium in the body, which is dependent upon the intensity of absorption and dilution. If absorption is speedy, it can pose a severe threat to the life of your pet.

In addition, many diseases to which our pets are vulnerable actually trigger the effects of fluid retention, and extraordinary thought should be given to ***drugs dispensed to pets*** that are inflicted with these diseases, as they are often a major reason for fluid retention.

Indications

Hyponatremia is manifested in several ways: lethargy-***slow response to your requests or demands***, polyuria, excessive drinking of water; seizures. These are foolproof signals that cannot be understated or ignored by pet owners. So, the first sign of lethargy should be promptly tested, as there could be a core problem that may be disguising itself. Extensive scans, neurological and blood tests must be administered to determine the most viable steps to take to protect the fitness of your pet.

A dog that has a heart failure can be at a serious health disadvantage when foods high in sodium cause sensitivity and discomfort to its stomach, and on skin and other areas of its body. Fluids can then be excessively built up in the body, causing the functioning of the heart to be undermined.

The perfect balance of sodium intake by pets can be accomplished in a meshing of concerted efforts of resources gained from clinical studies, combined with a methodical training system for pet owners, to greatly alleviate the agonies of this deficiency, or its profusion.

Relevant Links

www.petful.com

www.2ndchance.info.com

A Bit of Salty History

The Covenant of Salt is an ancient contract. It was a means of sealing an agreement between parties; for a loan, sale of goods, property, or for other legal matters.

Salt is essential to life; it heals, preserves, and, **as we know**, adds flavor and delight to food! People in ancient times appreciated its value, but we're not sure whether they were as cognizant as we are today of some of the health setbacks we endure when it's ingested in massive amounts.

As our civilization has developed over several years, we've searched and studied how to take advantage of the worth of sodium, and can now **manipulate** to what degree it affects our health.

When men had meals together, they became friends, since there was a strong connection between salt and promises. The Arabic expressions: "There is salt between us", and "He has eaten of my salt", were significant statements that implied a custom of pledge to friendship, and an everlasting covenant.

Another concept was that their **speech** had to be **seasoned with salt**; they had to say what they mean, and mean what they say.

And the custom among Arabic speaking people is still practiced. An Arab is bound by this custom to protect his most bitter enemy once he's eaten with him and while he's under his roof.

This explanation is not the main intention of this book; but only to show the significance, and diversity of its uses in certain cultures and, in a major way, in ***eating meals together.***

A more exhaustive study can be found online from ***multiple*** other sources!

www.truthortradition.com

An Endnote

When we find ourselves on the brink of having to make a decision that will impact our health and wellbeing, that's a great opportunity to go ahead and put aside all reasoning that may deter us from launching out and making the best possible choice.

We've seen our family, friends, and acquaintances endure maladies and even death, that could have been avoided by simply selecting the right foods. It seems too high a price to pay for daily ingesting the one mineral that can either hurt or help us, based on the quantity we consume.

Imagine! We don't have to agonize anymore when there are available resources to claim and apply so that we may enjoy an abundant life.

The sole reason for writing this book is this passion that I have for seeing people enjoying the best life they were created to live, without undue concerns about their fitness and that of their families and friends.

It's my heartfelt desire to know that people everywhere will be greatly helped by reading what I've shared from my personal experiences, and the research that I've done.

You can help me in my mission by leaving a review on Amazon and sharing your thoughts on this book. You have no idea how much this would help!

One last thing. How would you like winning **a \$200.00 Amazon Gift Card** and helping me improve this book in the process with a little bit of feedback?

That's right :)

Your opinion is so valuable to me that I am giving away a \$200 gift card to the luckiest *one of 200 participants*!

It will only take a minute of your time to let me know what you like and what you didn't like about this book. The hardest part is deciding how to spend the two hundred dollars!

Just follow this link.

http://booksfor.review/lowsodium